MASTERING RECOVERY FROM ADDICTION

Building Resilience

And Understanding

The Brain

To Overcome Addiction

Lovy Adams

TABLE OF CONTENTS

INTRODUCTION

The Path to Recovery Mastery

Starting the road to recovery takes a tremendous amount of courage and commitment. It is a route that can lead not only to addiction recovery but also to a better understanding of oneself and the possibility of a more fulfilled life. "MASTERING RECOVERY FROM ADDICTION: Building Resilience and Understanding the Brain to Overcome Addiction" is a handbook for people who are ready to embark on this life-changing journey.

Recovery is neither a linear nor a rapid fix. Instead, it is a lifelong quest for balance, health, and well-being. This book is based on the idea that by developing resilience and understanding the complicated workings of the brain, people can get the strength and knowledge needed to maintain a long-term recovery.

The science of addiction is complex, encompassing a tangle of elements that influence the development and function of the brain. This book delves into the neuroscience of addiction to provide a window into how narcotics and obsessive behaviors can hijack the brain's natural reward circuits, and more crucially, how these processes can be reversed.

A good recovery is built on resilience. It is a trait that enables people to overcome hardship, adapt to change, and emerge stronger. Throughout the book, readers will discover how to create resilience in a variety of forms—mental, emotional, and physical—giving them the tools they need to overcome the hurdles of recovery.

Each chapter is intended to provide useful ideas and insights that may be utilized in everyday life. From cognitive-behavioral approaches to mindfulness and meditation, lifestyle adjustments to relapse prevention, and the advice provided here is both evidence-based and user-friendly.

As recovery is a deeply personal path, this book recognizes the uniqueness of each person's experience. It promotes self-discovery and compassion, reminding readers that setbacks are not failures but rather opportunities for growth and learning.

You will also find stories of resilience—real-life experiences from folks who have walked the path of recovery—on these pages. These stories serve as beacons of hope, demonstrating that recovery is possible no matter how arduous the journey appears.

"Mastering Recovery from Addiction" is more than just a book; it is a companion for individuals who want to recover their lives from addiction. It is an invitation to engage on a journey that extends beyond sobriety, toward a life enriched by resilience, comprehension, and a restored sense of purpose.

Remember that you are not alone as you embark on this path. This book, as well as the community of those who have gone before you, is here to encourage and guide you every step of the road. Welcome to your path to recovery mastery.

CHAPTER ONE

The Nature of Addiction

Addiction and the Brain

Addiction is a complicated brain illness marked by compulsive substance use in the face of negative consequences. It is a disorder that can take over a person's life, influencing their behavior, relationships, and overall well-being. Addiction, at its foundation, includes basic alterations in the chemistry and function of the brain.

The brain that has been hijacked by substances or behaviors that increase the release of dopamine, a neurotransmitter associated with pleasure and reward is said to be addictive. The brain's reward system gradually changes, requiring more of the addictive substance or behavior to attain the same amount of satisfaction or "high." This section will look at the brain regions that are affected by addiction, the role of neurotransmitters, and the long-term effects of substance abuse on neural circuits.

Addiction has a substantial influence on the brain's structure and function. Addictive chemicals affect several critical brain regions, and understanding these areas can help explain why addiction is so powerful and difficult to escape.

Brain Regions Affected by Addiction:

The Reward System (containing the Ventral Tegmental Area (VTA), Nucleus Accumbens, and Prefrontal Cortex): This system is critical in the development of addiction. Dopamine, a neurotransmitter associated with pleasure, is released by the VTA into the nucleus accumbens, sometimes known as the brain's "pleasure center." The prefrontal cortex, which is in charge of decision-making and impulse control, is also implicated, which influences a person's capacity to resist desires.

The Amygdala and the Extended Amygdala: These areas are involved in tension and anxiety, which can be heightened during withdrawal and lead to a person seeking respite through substance use.

The Hippocampus: This area is linked to memory and learning. It aids in the formation of memories of the euphoria and pleasure associated with substance use, which can contribute to seeking and compulsive behavior.

Role of Neurotransmitters:

Dopamine: Known as the "feel-good" neurotransmitter, dopamine is essential in the reward circuit. Most addictive substances cause an increase in dopamine release or activity, which reinforces the act of using the substance.

Glutamate: A neurotransmitter required for learning and memory.

Changes in glutamate signaling can have an impact on reward-related learning processes, leading to the development of habitual substance seeking.

GABA (Gamma-Aminobutyric Acid): GABA is an inhibitory neurotransmitter that can be altered by substance usage, particularly benzodiazepines and alcohol. Changes in GABA function can impair impulse control, making it more difficult to resist cravings.

Serotonin: This neurotransmitter controls mood and some substances can change their action, contributing to mood swings and emotional difficulties that accompany addiction.

Long-Term Effects on Brain Pathways:

Substance abuse can cause long-term changes in the brain pathways, affecting behavior and cognition. These modifications include:

- Neuroplasticity Alterations: Substance use can hijack the brain's ability to adapt and reorganize itself, boosting the neural pathways linked with addiction while weakening those associated with non-addictive behaviors.
- Tolerance and Dependence: When a substance is used repeatedly, the brain adjusts to the excess dopamine by decreasing dopamine production or the number of dopamine receptors. This results in tolerance, in which more of the substance is required to achieve the same effect, and dependence, in which the brain depends on the substance to operate normally.
- Impaired Executive Function: Chronic substance use can harm the prefrontal cortex, decreasing a person's capacity to make decisions, control impulses, and regulate emotions, all of which are necessary for managing addictive behaviors.
- Withdrawal and Sensitization: Withdrawal symptoms are caused by the brain's response to the lack of the substance, whereas sensitization is the heightened response to a substance after repeated exposure, which increases the likelihood of relapse.

Recovery from addiction frequently entails treating these long-term changes through a variety of therapies that promote a healthy brain adaptation, aid in the re-establishment of neurotransmitter balance, and improve cognitive and emotional stability.

Addiction's Psychological Aspects

While understanding the scientific mechanisms of addiction is important, the psychosocial elements are also important. Addiction is frequently associated with a variety of psychological issues, such as emotional suffering, stress, and trauma. These issues can lead to people using substances as a coping mechanism. We will look at the psychological causes of addiction, such as anxiety, despair, and past traumas, in this section of the chapter. We will also look at how cognitive distortions and dysfunctional thought processes might contribute to the addiction cycle. Understanding these psychological components is essential for establishing effective healing solutions.

Psychological triggers are important in the development and maintenance of addiction. These triggers are inextricably linked to an individual's emotional and mental health experiences. Anxiety, depression, and past traumas are some of the most frequent psychological causes that can lead to substance use as people seek solace or escape from their problems.

Anxiety: People who suffer from anxiety may turn to drugs or alcohol to self-medicate and relieve their symptoms. The short respite afforded by narcotics can establish a self-perpetuating loop in which the individual continues to use in an attempt to manage anxiety, eventually leading to addiction.

Depression: Those suffering from depression may also use substances to numb their misery or hopelessness. The first "lift" provided by drugs or alcohol may appear to be a remedy for their bad mood.

Substance abuse, on the other hand, can increase depression over time, especially as the effects wear off and withdrawal sets in.

Past Traumas: Traumatic events, such as abuse, accidents, or loss, can leave emotional scars that last a lifetime. Individuals who have unresolved trauma may use drugs or alcohol to avoid painful memories or emotions related to these events. This avoidance can obstruct trauma processing and recovery, leading to a reliance on substances for emotional regulation.

Cognitive distortions are incorrect thought patterns that can contribute to the addiction cycle. These are some examples:

All-or-Nothing Thinking: Thinking in black-and-white terms about situations. For example, a person may assume that one blunder implies they have failed totally, leading to chronic substance abuse.

Overgeneralization is the process of drawing broad inferences from a particular occurrence. An individual may see a poor day as proof that life will always be horrible unless they utilize narcotics.

Catastrophizing is the expectation that the worst-case the situation will occur. This might result in heightened anxiety and the perception of a need for narcotics to cope with impending disaster.

Minimization refers to downplaying the negative repercussions of substance use or one's ability to quit, which might delay seeking treatment.

Maladaptive cognitive patterns are habitual methods of thinking that are frequently negative and counterproductive. These are some examples:

Self-Medication: Believing that drugs or alcohol are required to cope with stress, emotions, or mental health problems.

Denial is the refusal to recognize the negative repercussions of substance usage on one's life and health.

Making justifications for substance usage or blaming external conditions for one's actions is referred to as rationalization.

Helplessness: The feeling of being powerless to change one's situation or conduct, which leads to continuous substance use as a coping mechanism.

By sustaining the assumption that substance use is the legitimate solution to emotional and psychological anguish, these cognitive distortions and maladaptive thought processes can perpetuate the cycle of addiction.

Overcoming these tendencies necessitates a mix of self-awareness, cognitive-behavioral tactics, and, in many cases, professional assistance in developing healthy ways of thinking and coping with life's obstacles.

The Addiction Cycle

Addiction is not a static condition; it is a cyclical process that might be difficult to overcome. The addiction cycle often begins with experimentation or voluntary use and progresses to regular use, tolerance, and dependence. When individuals become dependent, they may experience withdrawal symptoms when attempting to quit, leading to continuing use to soothe discomfort, thus perpetuating the cycle.

This section will go over the stages of the addiction cycle, such as first use, abuse, dependence, and relapse. Recognizing the patterns inside this cycle is the first step toward breaking it and moving on. We will also go over the elements that can cause a relapse and how to prepare for and respond to them.

The addiction cycle is a complicated process that usually progresses through numerous stages, each with its own set of obstacles and behaviors.

Understanding these stages can aid in spotting the signs of addiction and implementing effective recovery and relapse prevention techniques.

Initial Use: The cycle frequently begins with the first use of a substance. Curiosity, peer pressure, or an attempt to self-medicate emotional distress may all be factors. For some, this stage consists of experimenting with no progression to further use. For others, however, the first use can set the foundation for a pattern of behavior that develops into addiction.

Abuse: The individual's substance usage becomes more frequent or intense throughout this stage. They may begin to use substances in greater quantities or in more unsafe situations, such as while driving. The individual's substance use begins to have negative effects on his or her life, such as problems with relationships, employment, or education, but the usage persists despite these challenges.

Dependence: Dependence is defined by the urge to continue using the substance in order to avoid withdrawal symptoms and to feel "normal."

Tolerance occurs when the body has adapted to the presence of the substance and requires more of it to get the desired effect. Dependence can be either psychological or physical.

Relapse: Relapse is the return to substance usage following a period of abstinence. It is a normal component of the rehabilitation process and does not imply failure; rather, it emphasizes the need for continued or modified treatment measures.

A relapse can be precipitated by a number of circumstances, including:

- Stress: Excessive stress might cause a desire to escape or relieve tension through substance abuse.
- Environmental Cues: Places, people, or things connected with previous substance use might elicit strong cravings.
- Negative Emotional States: Sadness, loneliness, worry, or boredom can lead to a return to substance use as a coping technique.
- Peer Pressure: Peer pressure or social contexts where substance use might lead to relapse.
- Complacency: Being overconfident in one's capacity to resist urges or underestimating the power of addiction can lead to a drop in guard and a potential relapse.

Consider the following techniques to prepare for and respond to these challenges:

- Create a Support System: Engage with friends, relatives, or support groups that understand the recovery journey and can provide encouragement and aid when confronted with triggers.
- Study Stress Management Methods: To manage stress without resorting to substance abuse, try relaxing techniques such as deep breathing, meditation, or exercise.
- Avoid High-Risk Situations: Recognize and avoid places or persons who may heighten the desire to use substances.
- Develop a Relapse Prevention Plan: Work with a therapist or counselor to create a specific plan that includes coping methods for cravings and triggers.
- Seek Professional Help: If you're worried about relapsing, seek help from a healthcare provider, therapist, or addiction expert.
- Practice Self-Care: Make sure you are taking care of your physical and emotional health by eating well, exercising, sleeping well, and engaging in enjoyable activities.
- Gain Knowledge through Experience: If you relapse, consider what happened and why. Use this information to improve your relapse prevention strategy and make positive changes to your recovery strategy.

Remember that recovery is a journey, and relapse does not indicate the end. It's an opportunity to learn, grow, and keep striving toward a drug-free lifestyle.

CHAPTER TWO

The Science of the Brain

This chapter delves into the complex workings of the brain, investigating the neuroscience of addiction, the phenomena of neuroplasticity in recovery, and the essential role neurotransmitters play in these processes.

Addiction Neurobiology

Addiction is a complicated brain illness marked by compulsive substance use in the face of negative consequences. The brain's reward system, which is hijacked by addictive chemicals, lies at the heart of addiction. When a person uses a drug, their brain produces a rush of dopamine, rewarding drug-related actions by establishing a strong loop of bliss and yearning.

Addiction disrupts the brain's circuitry, resulting in alterations in the function of the prefrontal cortex, which inhibits decision-making and self-control. The amygdala becomes hypersensitive to the presence of the drug, and the hippocampus forms powerful memories connected with the drug experience, which further entrenches the addiction.

Neuroplasticity and Rehabilitation

Neuroplasticity refers to the brain's amazing ability to remodel and develop new neural connections throughout life. This flexibility is essential not just for learning and memory, but also for addiction rehabilitation.

As a person abstains from substance use throughout recovery, their brain begins to mend. Addiction-destructive habits can be replaced with new, healthy patterns of behavior and mental processes. Therapy, social support, exercise, and mindfulness can all promote positive neuroplasticity, restoring brain balance and lowering the chance of recurrence.

The Function of Neurotransmitters

Neurotransmitters are chemical messengers in the brain that convey impulses between neurons (nerve cells), which govern every aspect of human function, from breathing to thinking to feeling.

Dopamine is not the only neurotransmitter that has a role in addiction. Glutamate, the primary excitatory neurotransmitter, is required for learning and memory, as well as for the creation of desires and the reinforcement of the addiction cycle. GABA, the primary inhibitory neurotransmitter, helps to regulate excitability and is commonly disrupted in addiction, leading to anxiety and impaired impulse control.

Another major neurotransmitter that impacts mood is serotonin, which is frequently targeted by drugs such as MDMA (ecstasy) and some medications. Serotonin imbalances can lead to mood problems, which frequently co-occur with addiction.

Understanding the science of the brain is critical for creating successful addiction therapies and assisting individuals on their road to recovery. It is possible to break the hold of addiction and live a healthy, full life by leveraging the power of neuroplasticity and harmonizing neurotransmitters.

CHAPTER THREE

Assessing Your Own Path

Self-awareness is a critical component in the recovery from addiction path. This chapter will assist you in assessing your personal recovery route, with an emphasis on identifying the need for change, engaging in self-assessment and reflection, and setting intentions that will lead you to resilience and healing.

Awareness of the Need for Change

The first step in any healing process is to admit that change is required. This is frequently followed by the realization that substance use has become destructive, resulting in poor effects on health, relationships, jobs, or legal status. Recognizing the need for change is a courageous and critical first step in recovery.

Addiction Signs and Symptoms

Addiction manifests itself through a variety of indications and symptoms that can damage physical, psychological, and social aspects of life.

These might include:

- Desire for the substance
- Increased tolerance, needing more of the substance to produce the same effect
- Withdrawal symptoms when not using the substance
- Loss of control over the quantity and frequency of use
- Neglecting obligations at home, work, or school
- Giving up previously loved hobbies

- Engaging in unsafe actions while under the influence
- Relationship issues caused by substance abuse

Recognizing these indications and symptoms in oneself or others might be the first step in getting assistance.

Substance Abuse's Consequences

Substance misuse may have far-reaching implications for many aspects of life:

Health issues ranging from short-term effects to chronic diseases or overdose

Mental health issues such as depression, anxiety, and psychosis

- Financial difficulties due to the cost of obtaining substances and decreased productivity
- Legal issues such as arrest, incarceration, and a criminal record
- Damaged relationships with family, friends, and colleagues
- Social isolation and stigma
- Impaired cognitive abilities and brain function

These implications highlight the need to treat drug misuse as a serious problem that requires help.

Accepting Addiction's Reality

Acceptance is an important stage in the healing process. It entails admitting that substance abuse has become a problem in one's life and that assistance is required to overcome it. Acceptance can be tough since it entails addressing uncomfortable realities and feelings. It is, however, empowering since it is the first step toward making positive changes.

Acceptance entails:

- Recognizing the impact of addiction on you and others lives
- Recognizing addiction as an illness that affects the brain and behavior;
- Being open to the notion of treatment and recovery;
- Committing to the recovery process, even when it is tough; and

- Seeking help from experts, peers, and loved ones.
- Accepting the truth of addiction is the cornerstone of a successful recovery, leading to a road of healing and a more satisfying life.

Self-Evaluation and Reflection

After recognizing the need for change, the next stage is to examine the inside. Examining your drug use habits, triggers, and the underlying causes of your addiction are all part of self-assessment. Understanding the impact of your addiction on your life and the lives of people around you is the goal of reflection.

Identifying Substance Use Patterns

Recognizing patterns in drug usage is a necessary step in comprehending the nature of one's addiction. The frequency and quantity of drug use, certain times of the day or social contexts when use happens, and the sorts of substances used are all examples of patterns. It also entails recognizing the addiction cycle, such as times of high use followed by attempts to quit or restrict usage, as well as probable relapses. Individuals can begin to see the routine nature of their behavior and the conditions that contribute to their substance use by recognizing these patterns.

Recognizing Triggers and Cravings

Triggers are particular stimuli that cause drug use urges, which are strong wants to use substances. External triggers, such as locations, people, or events connected with previous substance use, might be external, or internal, such as emotions or stress. Cravings are frequently the result of a physiological and psychological reaction to certain cues. Understanding one's specific triggers and the ensuing cravings is critical for creating coping mechanisms that do not include substance use.

Investigating Subsequent Emotional and Psychological Factors

Many people use drugs to cope with emotional anguish, stress, or trauma. Exploring the underlying emotional and psychological issues that lead to addiction is a difficult process that frequently needs expert assistance. It entails digging into one's background, recognizing problematic thought patterns, and addressing any co-occurring mental health conditions.

Individuals can begin to address the basic reasons for their addiction and establish healthy coping methods by identifying these underlying elements.

Evaluating the Effects on Your Life and Relationships

Substance addiction may have serious consequences for one's physical health, emotional well-being, work performance, and financial stability. Relationships with family, friends, and coworkers may suffer as well. Assessing this influence entails looking at the implications of substance use and realizing how it has hampered one's capacity to live a full life.

Because it emphasizes the significance of healing in restoring a sense of formality and mending damaged relationships, this evaluation may be a powerful incentive for change.

Setting Recovery Intentions

You may begin to create objectives for your recovery after you have a firm grasp of your addiction and its repercussions. Intentions differ from objectives in that they include committing to a process and accepting that recovery is a journey with ups and downs. Intention setting entails clarifying what resilience and recovery mean to you and how you want to attain them.

Making a Recovery Vision

Your recovery vision is a personal and vivid depiction of how you want your life to be without the impact of addiction. It encapsulates your beliefs, aims, and aspirations and acts as a motivating guidepost.

Consider what is most important to you while defining your vision, such as your health, relationships, job, or personal growth. Consider how you want to feel, the activities you want to do, and the connections you want to develop or restore. Your recovery vision should both inspire and remind you of why you are dedicated to this transformational journey.

How to Develop a Resilient Mindset

A resilient mentality is essential for handling the difficulties and setbacks that may arise throughout rehabilitation. It entails building a persevering, adaptable, and optimistic mindset. To develop a resilient attitude, practice self-compassion, focus on your strengths, and maintain a growth mindset that sees setbacks as chances to learn. Building resilience also entails creating a support network and learning to ask for help when it is required. You can confront obstacles with confidence and remain committed to rehabilitation even while under stress if you have resilience.

Creating a Personal Recovery Plan

A personalized recovery plan is a customized blueprint that details the particular measures you will take to attain your recovery goal. It should take into account your specific circumstances, such as your history of substance abuse, personal strengths and limitations, and life obligations. Your treatment approach may include therapy, medication-assisted treatment, support groups, and lifestyle modifications such as exercise and diet. It should also contain techniques for dealing with triggers and cravings, as well as contingency plans for probable relapses.

Determining Short-Term and Long-Term Goals

Setting intentions, both short-term and long-term, is a good method to sketch out your recovery path. Short-term goals might include going to a particular number of support group sessions each week, practicing mindfulness every day, or abstaining from substances for a month. Long-term objectives may include healing relationships, fulfilling job goals, or being sober for a year or longer. To maximize the chance of success, these objectives should be precise, measurable, attainable, relevant, and time-bound (SMART). They give structure and responsibility, allowing you to focus on the tasks required to advance toward your wider recovery objective.

CHAPTER FOUR

Cultivating Mental Resilience

Mental resilience is the inner strength that allows people to bounce back from setbacks and stay on the path to sobriety during their recovery journey. This chapter dives into the notion of resilience, presents ways for building it, and offers guidance on how to retain resilience when confronted with cravings.

How to Understand Resilience

Resilience is the psychological attribute that permits people to be knocked down by life's difficulties and recover at least as strongly as they were before. Rather than allowing failure to deplete their determination, they find a way to rise from the ashes. Resilience is not a feature that people either have or do not have in the context of addiction treatment. It involves attitudes, ideas, and actions that everyone may acquire and grow.

Resilience's Role in Recovery

Resilience is essential in the rehabilitation of addiction. Individuals' inner strength is what allows them to navigate the inevitable hurdles and setbacks that occur along the rehabilitation process. Individuals with resilience are able to sustain their focus on sobriety in the face of cravings, triggers, and the stress of life transitions. It also enables people to learn from gaps or mistakes instead of getting sidetracked by them. Individuals who are resilient are better suited to manage the emotional and psychological work involved in recovery, and they are more likely to maintain their sobriety over time.

The Science of Resilience

The psychology of resilience is based on a person's capacity to cope with stress and hardship. This coping ability entails cognitive, emotional, and behavioral adaptability. Resilient people tend to have a more optimistic attitude in life, with a strong conviction in their own abilities to handle their emotions. They regard challenges as transient and malleable rather than permanent and intractable. Self-esteem, optimism, and a feeling of purpose or meaning in life are all components of the psychological framework of resilience. These characteristics all contribute to an individual's ability to recover and even flourish from adversity.

Learning to be Resilient

While some people are born with more resilient qualities than others, resilience is a skill that can be taught and reinforced over time. Adopting a set of skills and attitudes that may be practiced and incorporated into daily life is part of learning resilience. Problem-solving, communication, and emotional control are all skills that may be refined via therapy, self-reflection, and real-world experiences. Fostering supportive relationships and searching out strong role models can also help to boost resilience. Individuals in recovery empower themselves to actively enhance their capacity to tolerate and recover from setbacks by perceiving resilience as a skill set that can be expanded.

Strategies for Increasing Resilience

Building resilience is a personal journey with no one-size-fits-all solution. However, there are various ways that might help you deal with the stresses of recovery:

- Establishing a Strong Support Network: It is critical to surround oneself with understanding individuals in order to create resilience.
- Embracing Change: Flexibility is an important component of resilience. Being more adaptive might help you deal with the unpredictability of rehabilitation.
- Practicing Positive Thinking: Optimism is an important component of resilience. While you do not have to disregard reality, a positive attitude will allow you to deal with difficult situations more effectively.

- Concentrating on What You Can Control: You can feel more empowered and confident in your recovery path by focusing on your own actions and habits.
- Maintaining Your Physical Health: Physical and mental health are inextricably intertwined. Resilience may be improved by exercise, a healthy diet, and enough sleep.

Stability in the Face of Cravings

Cravings are a natural part of recovery and can be difficult to overcome, but resilience can help you avoid the temptation to relapse. Here are some strategies for becoming resilient during difficult times:

- Mindfulness and meditation: These techniques can help you become more aware of your urges and manage them without succumbing to them.
- Cognitive Restructuring: Changing your thinking about desires can help to diminish their potency. Instead of viewing hunger as a sign of weakness, consider it a chance to build your resilience.
- Delaying Tactics: When a craving strikes, postpone acting on it. If you wait long enough, the impulse will usually pass.
- Distraction Techniques: Engaging in a hobby, exercise, or any other activity that you love helps divert your attention away from the urge.
- Reflecting on Past Successes: Remind yourself of previous occasions when you successfully handled urges. This might enhance your confidence and assist you in overcoming existing obstacles.

CHAPTER FIVE

Emotional Resilience in Recovery

Building emotional resilience is essential for long-term addiction rehabilitation. This chapter looks at how people may regulate their emotions without using narcotics, improve their emotional intelligence, and use methods for emotional regulation.

Emotional Management without Substances

Many people use narcotics as a coping method to deal with negative feelings. It is critical in recovery to find alternate strategies to deal with these feelings:

- Recognizing and Naming Emotions: Recognize and identify your emotions in order to understand what you are experiencing and why.
- Acceptance: Recognize and accept your feelings without judgment. Recognize that having a wide variety of emotions is natural.
- Seeking Help: Talk to friends, relatives, or support groups about your emotional experiences to obtain perspective.
- Healthy Outlets: Use hobbies such as exercise, painting, or writing to manage emotions in a healthy way.

Emotional Intelligence Development

Emotional intelligence (EI) is the capacity to identify and affect the emotions of others as well as comprehend and regulate your own.

Developing EI can help with healing significantly:

- Self-awareness: Be aware of your emotional condition and how it influences your ideas and actions.
- Self-regulation: Develop the ability to regulate impulsive sentiments and behaviors, manage your emotions in healthy ways, and take initiative.
- Motivation: Direct your emotions toward a goal, which in the context of recovery is sobriety maintenance.
- Empathy: Understanding the feelings of others helps enhance communication and relationships, both of which are critical components of a support network.
- Social Skills: Enhance your capacity to speak clearly, lead people, and handle conflict, which is very useful in group recovery situations

Emotional Regulation Tools

Emotional regulation is the capacity to control and respond appropriately to an emotional event. Several tools can be used to improve emotional regulation:

- Being mindful Meditation is practicing being present in the moment and notice your feelings objectively.
- Deep breathing techniques can help to soothe the nervous system and lessen stress.
- Cognitive Behavioral Therapy (CBT): Use CBT strategies to question and modify problematic thought patterns and behaviors.
- Dialectical Behavior Therapy (DBT): Use DBT methods to manage stress, control emotions, and improve interpersonal relationships.
- Progressive Muscle Relaxation: This technique relieves physical tension in the body, which is typically associated with powerful emotions.

CHAPTER SIX

Physical Resilience and Well-being

Physical resilience and well-being are equally crucial in the recovery process as psychological elements.This chapter focuses on the significance of physical health in long-term rehabilitation, the benefits of exercise as a recovery strategy, and the effect of diet on brain function.

The Importance of Physical Fitness

Physical health serves as the basis for emotional and mental resiliency. Substance misuse may have a substantial impact on the body, and rehabilitation provides an opportunity to restore and strengthen one's physical condition. Improving physical health can result in a better overall mood, more energy, and a greater capacity to cope with stress. It might also act as a daily reminder of one's resolve to live a better, drug-free life.

Rebuilding the Body: Post-Addiction Body Healing Strategies

Rebuilding the body after addiction entails a multifaceted strategy for regaining physical health and overall well-being. It usually includes:

1. Dietary Guidelines: Malnutrition is a common result of substance addiction. A nutritious diet high in vitamins, minerals, and antioxidants is essential. Incorporating entire meals such as fruits, vegetables, lean meats, and whole grains can aid in bodily healing and immune system enhancement.

2. Hydration: Water is vital for flushing away toxins, supporting renal function, and maintaining general physiological functioning.

3. Exercise: Regular physical exercise can enhance cardiovascular health, muscle strength, endorphin release to improve mood, and stress reduction. Exercise can also aid in the establishment of a healthy routine.

4. Medical Care: To treat any long-term health difficulties created by addiction, ongoing medical care may be required. Treatment for liver disease, infections, or other organ damage might be included.

5. Mental Health Support: Therapy and counseling can aid in the recovery process and avoid relapse by addressing the psychological components of addiction.

Sleep and Recovery: Understanding Sleep's Restorative Power

Sleep aids in the recovery from addiction by:

1. Healing:

The body restores itself during sleep. This includes restoring brain function and fortifying the immune system.

2. Emotional Regulation: Adequate sleep aids in the regulation of emotions and the improvement of mood, which is especially essential for those in recovery who may experience mood fluctuations or emotional discomfort.

3. Cognitive Function: Sleep is essential for cognitive activities including memory, attention, and decision-making, all of which can be hampered by addiction.

4. Stress Reduction: Sleep aids in the reduction of stress hormone levels in the body, which might otherwise cause cravings and relapse.

5. Habit Formation: Creating a regular sleep pattern can aid in the formation of other healthy habits, which are an important component of the recovery process.

Physical Withdrawal Management: Techniques for Coping with Withdrawal Physical Symptoms

Managing physical withdrawal requires numerous tactics, including:

1. Medical Detox: Medication and assistance can be provided by a supervised detox program to properly treat withdrawal symptoms.

2. Hydration and Nutrition: Keeping fluid intake and nutrition balance will help relieve certain withdrawal symptoms.

3. Relaxation Techniques: Deep breathing, meditation, and progressive muscle relaxation a techniques that can help you manage stress and discomfort.

4. Distraction: Activities such as reading, listening to music, or mild exercise might help to distract from withdrawal symptoms.

5. Support Networks: A robust support network of friends, family, or support groups can give encouragement and lessen feelings of loneliness during withdrawal.

6. Expert Assistance: Consulting with a healthcare expert can give advice on the best strategies for dealing with withdrawal and preparing for long-term recovery.

Exercise as a Tool for Recovery

Exercise is an extremely effective rehabilitation technique.It can help you arrange your day, minimize stress, and enhance your mental health outcomes.

In this book, the connection between physical activity and recovery is a key focus, particularly in how exercise can lead to natural endorphin release, stress reduction, and the establishment of routine and discipline.

Natural Endorphin Release: How Physical Activity Improves Mood and Decreases Anxiety and Despair

Exercise is a powerful trigger for the release of endorphins, the body's natural feel-good chemicals. These endorphins interact with the receptors in the brain that reduce the perception of pain and trigger a positive feeling in the body, often referred to as a "runner's high."

Here's how physical activity leverages endorphin release to improve mood and mental health:

- Regular physical activity increases endorphin levels, which can lead to improved mood and a sense of well-being.

- Exercise can act as a natural anti-anxiety treatment by reducing stress hormones and releasing endorphins.

- Physical activity can help alleviate symptoms of depression by promoting neural growth, reducing inflammation, and fostering feelings of calm and well-being.

Stress Reduction: The Importance of Exercise in Stress Management and Its Impact on Relapse Prevention

Stress is a common trigger for relapse in individuals recovering from addiction. Exercise plays a vital role in managing stress for several reasons:

- It reduces levels of the body's stress hormones, such as adrenaline and cortisol, which can be elevated during recovery.

- Exercise stimulates the production of endorphins, which not only reduce pain but also counteract stress and enhance mood.

- Physical activity provides a healthy outlet for frustration and tension, which can build up during the recovery process.

- Regular exercise has been associated with improved sleep patterns, which can be disrupted by stress and are crucial for overall stress management.

By incorporating exercise into the recovery process, individuals can better manage stress, which in turn can reduce the risk of relapse.

Routine and Discipline: How Regular Exercise May Help You Develop Positive Habits and Self-Discipline

Exercise can be a powerful tool for establishing a routine and discipline, which is essential for a successful recovery journey:

- Structured exercise routines provide a sense of purpose and order, which can be particularly grounding for individuals in recovery.

- The discipline necessary to maintain a regular exercise routine can be transferred to other aspects of life, producing a better sense of control and self-efficacy.

- As exercise becomes a habitual part of one's lifestyle, it can replace the negative habits associated with addiction, providing a positive and healthful alternative.

- The commitment to regular physical activity can reinforce the commitment to recovery, as both require ongoing effort and dedication.

In summary, by engaging in regular physical activity, individuals in recovery can experience natural endorphin release, effective stress management, and the development of a disciplined routine, all of which contribute to a more resilient and successful recovery process.

Nutrition and Cognitive Function

To operate properly, the brain requires a variety of nutrients, many of which can be reduced by substance addiction. A proper diet can aid in brain repair and cognitive function, all of which are required for a full recovery.

The interaction between diet, brain chemistry, and recovery is a vital component that may dramatically affect an individual's sober path.

Brain Chemistry and Nutrition: How Different Nutrients Affect Mood and Addiction Neurotransmitters

- Nutrition has a significant influence on brain chemistry, particularly neurotransmitters, which are chemical messengers involved in mood regulation and addiction. As an example:

- Amino acids, present in protein-rich diets, are precursors to neurotransmitters related to pleasure and well-being, including dopamine and serotonin.

Getting enough protein can help balance these neurotransmitters.

- Omega-3 fatty acids, which are found in fish, flaxseeds, and walnuts, are important for brain health and have been demonstrated to boost mood and cognitive performance.

- Whole-grain complex carbs help balance blood sugar levels, which can help reduce mood swings and boost the availability of tryptophan in the brain, which is a precursor to serotonin.

- Vitamins and minerals, including B vitamins, vitamin D, magnesium, and zinc are essential for neurotransmitter production and activity.

Anti-inflammatory Foods: The Health Benefits of Reducing Inflammation in the Brain and Body

Chronic inflammation can harm both the body and the brain, possibly aggravating mood problems and impeding recovery. Anti-inflammatory foods can aid in the reduction of inflammation:

- Fruits and vegetables, particularly leafy greens and berries, are high in anti-inflammatory antioxidants and phytonutrients.

- Turmeric and ginger include chemicals that are anti-inflammatory.

- Omega-3 fatty acid-rich foods, such as fatty fish, have been found to lower inflammation in the brain, potentially improving mental health and cognitive performance.

Recovery Meal Planning: Tips for Incorporating a Balanced Diet into a Recovery Plan

A well-balanced diet is critical for supplying the body with the nutrients it requires to recuperate. Here are some meal-planning suggestions:

- Aim for regular, balanced meals throughout the day to maintain energy levels and mood stability.

- Eat a variety of foods to get a wide spectrum of nutrients. Each meal should have a healthy mix of proteins, carbs, and fats.

- Drink lots of water to stay hydrated, which is important for general health and can help curb cravings.

- Plan and prepare meals ahead of time to limit the chances of impulsive eating or relying on less nutritional alternatives.

- Be conscious of your eating patterns, acknowledging that recovery might be a time when food is used to replace drugs.

Concentrate on eating for nutrition and wellness.

Individuals in recovery can support their brain's healing process, reduce cravings, and improve their overall well-being as they work towards long-term sobriety by understanding and applying brain chemistry and nutrition principles, incorporating anti-inflammatory foods, and strategically planning meals.

CHAPTER SEVEN

Cognitive Approaches to Recovery

This chapter explores the cognitive approaches to recovery, focusing on Cognitive Behavioral Therapy (CBT), the process of challenging and changing thoughts, and the application of mindfulness in the context of recovery.

Cognitive Behavioral Therapy (CBT) Basics

Cognitive Behavioral Therapy is a widely used therapeutic approach that helps individuals identify and change negative thought patterns and behaviors. In the context of addiction recovery, CBT can be particularly effective in tackling the cognitive distortions that often contribute to substance abuse. This section would cover:

The Theory behind CBT: Understanding How Thoughts, Feelings, and Behaviorsare interconnected

The theory behind Cognitive Behavioral Therapy (CBT) is founded on the principle that our thoughts, feelings, and behaviors are intricately linked and influence one another. According to CBT, negative and dysfunctional thoughts can lead to distressing emotions and maladaptive behaviors, which can then reinforce negative thinking. In the context of recovery, understanding this cycle is crucial because substance abuse is often a behavior that's influenced by negative thought patterns and feelings.

By learning to identify and understand these negative thoughts, individuals can begin to challenge and modify them, which can lead to changes in emotions and behaviors. For example, if someone believes they cannot cope with stress without using substances (a thought), they may feel hopeless (an emotion) and reach for drugs or alcohol as a coping mechanism (a behavior). CBT aims to break this cycle by providing tools to change the thought, which in turn can change the feeling and the behavior.

CBT Techniques

CBT offers a range of techniques that can help individuals change their thought patterns and behaviors:

- Cognitive Restructuring: This technique involves identifying and challenging negative and irrational thoughts, and replacing them with more balanced and realistic ones. For example, changing the thought "I will never be able to recover" to "Recovery is challenging, but I can take it one step at a time."

- Behavioral Activation: This strategy encourages individuals to engage in activities that they find enjoyable or fulfilling. The goal is to combat the inertia and withdrawal that often accompany depression and to reinforce positive behaviors that are incompatible with substance use.

- Exposure Therapy: This technique involves gradual exposure to feared situations or objects in a controlled and safe way. Over time, exposure helps reduce the fear and anxiety associated with these triggers. In addiction recovery, exposure therapy can be used to help individuals confront and manage cravings and triggers without relapse.

Goal Setting in CBT

Goal setting in CBT is an important aspect of the therapeutic process, as it provides direction and motivation. Here's how to set realistic and achievable goals in recovery:

- Specificity: Goals should be clear and specific. Instead of a vague goal like "get better," a specific goal might be "attend three support group meetings per week."

- Measurability: Goals should be measurable so that progress can be tracked. For instance, "reduce drinking episodes from four times a week to once a week."

- Achievability: Goals should be realistic and attainable. Setting goals that are too ambitious can lead to disappointment and a sense of failure.

- Relevance: Goals should be relevant to the individual's recovery and personal aspirations.

- Time-Bound: Goals should have a timeframe to provide a sense of urgency and a deadline for completion.

By setting goals in this manner, individuals can see tangible progress in their recovery journey, which can be incredibly motivating and reinforce of the positive changes they are making.

Challenging and Changing Thoughts

One of the core components of CBT is learning to challenge and change unhelpful thoughts. This process is crucial in recovery as it empowers individuals to shift their perspective and respond to situations in a healthier way. Topics might include:

Identifying Negative Thought Patterns

Recognizing common cognitive distortions is a fundamental step in Cognitive Behavioral Therapy (CBT) and self-improvement. These distortions are irrational or exaggerated thought patterns that can lead to negative emotions and behaviors. Some examples include:

- 'All-or-Nothing' Thinking: This is a pattern where you see things in black-and-white categories. If a situation falls short of perfect, you see it as a total failure. For example, if you slip up once on a diet, you might think, "I've blown it, I might as well give up."

- Overgeneralization: You might take a single negative event as a never-ending pattern of defeat. For instance, if something goes wrong at work, you think, "I always mess up" or "I'll never get it right."

- Catastrophizing: This involves expecting disaster to strike, no matter what. For example, you might worry excessively about making a small mistake on a project, thinking it will lead to a major catastrophe in your career.

The Power of Reframing

Reframing involves changing the way you perceive an event and thus changing your experience of it. Here are some techniques for reframing negative thoughts:

- Evidence-Based Thinking: Challenge your negative thoughts by looking for evidence against them. If you think "I always fail," list successes you've had to counter this belief.

- Alternative Viewpoint: Try to see the situation from someone else's perspective. Ask yourself, "What would my friend think about this situation? Would they see it as I do?"

- Outcome Exploration: Consider the best, worst, and most likely outcomes of the situation. Often, you'll find that the worst-case scenario is not as likely or catastrophic as you initially thought.

- Gratitude Focusing: Shift your focus to what's good in your life. This can help counterbalance the negativity bias that often accompanies distorted thinking.

Building Cognitive Resilience

The capacity to recover from setbacks and retain an optimistic view is referred to as cognitive resilience. Here are some methods for increasing cognitive resilience:

- Cognitive Flexibility: Practice looking at situations from multiple angles and being open to new information. This can help you adapt to changing circumstances.

- Problem-Solving Skills: Improve your problem-solving skills by breaking them down into smaller, more manageable chunks and addressing them one at a time.

- Positive Self-Talk: Encourage yourself with positive affirmations and compassionate self-talk, especially during challenging times.

- Stress Management Techniques: To retain a balanced viewpoint, engage in stress-relieving activities such as exercise, meditation, or hobbies.

You may cultivate a more positive mentality that promotes personal growth and recovery by detecting and confronting negative thinking patterns, mastering the art of reframing, and developing cognitive resilience.

Mindfulness and Mindful Recovery

Mindfulness is the discipline of being completely present and engaged in the present moment, conscious of one's thoughts and sensations but without judgment.

In recovery, mindfulness can be a valuable tool for maintaining focus on sobriety and managing cravings.

The Basics of Mindfulness: An Introduction to Mindfulness

Practices and Their Benefits

Mindfulness is the deliberate practice of concentrating one's attention on the present moment without judgment. It entails being fully aware of your current experiences, including thoughts, feelings, sensations, and your surroundings.

 The benefits of mindfulness are extensive and can include reduced stress, improved emotional regulation, enhanced cognitive flexibility, and a greater capacity for compassion and empathy.

Mindfulness activities urge people to notice their thoughts and feelings exactly as they are, without attempting to modify or evaluate them. This can result in a more in-depth awareness of oneself as well as a more welcoming and sympathetic attitude. Mindfulness can help people become more aware of their cravings and emotional triggers in the context of addiction treatment, allowing them to respond to these problems with more choice and self-control.

Mindfulness Meditation: Guided Exercises and Techniques to Foster Mindfulness

Mindfulness meditation is a key practice in developing mindfulness. Here are some guided exercises and techniques:

- Breath Awareness: This entails focusing on the natural rhythm of your breath. As you breathe in and out, you gently bring your focus back to your breath whenever your mind wanders. This simple practice can ground you in the present moment and calm the mind.

- Body Scan: Starting at the toes and moving upwards, you pay attention to each part of the body, noticing any sensations, tension, or discomfort. The body scan promotes a state of relaxation and body awareness, helping to release physical and mental tension.

- Mindful Observation: Choose an object and focus all your attention on it. Observe it objectively, noting its shape, color, texture, and other characteristics. This practice improves your capacity to focus and be totally present.

Applying Mindfulness in Recovery: Strategies for Using Mindfulness to Cope with Triggers, Reduce Stress, and Enhance Emotional Regulation

Incorporating mindfulness into recovery can be a powerful strategy for managing the challenges that come with overcoming addiction:

- Coping with Triggers: Mindfulness helps individuals recognize the early signs of craving and allows them to observe these triggers with detachment. By acknowledging cravings without acting on them, one can reduce their power.

- Reducing Stress: Mindfulness techniques, such as deep breathing and meditation can activate the body's relaxation response, countering the stress response that often accompanies and exacerbates addiction.

- Enhancing Emotional Regulation: Mindfulness encourages a non-reactive stance toward one's emotions. Over time, this practice helps individuals experience their emotions without being overwhelmed by them, leading to better emotional balance and resilience.

Individuals in recovery can develop crucial skills to help them stay focused on their objectives, handle unpleasant emotions and thoughts, and eventually lead a more balanced and satisfying life by practicing mindfulness.

CHAPTER EIGHT

Relapse Prevention Planning

Relapse prevention is an essential component of long-term rehabilitation. This chapter discusses recognizing triggers, developing a specific relapse prevention strategy, and dealing with impulses and cravings.

How to Recognize Triggers and High-Risk Situations

The first step in relapse prevention is identifying the exact triggers and high-risk scenarios that may lead to substance abuse. Triggers can be emotional, such as feelings of tension, anxiety, or depression. They can also be physical, such as visiting a location where one used to participate in substance use, or social, such as being in the company of people who use substances. High-risk environments are ones that increase the likelihood of relapse, such as social gatherings, stressful events, or even specific times of the day or week.

Individuals can successfully detect triggers and high-risk circumstances by:

- Reflecting on prior experiences to spot patterns that have led to substance use.

- Keep track of sensations, thoughts, and actions that occur before cravings.

- Seek advice from therapists, support groups, or trustworthy friends who can help you identify possible triggers.

Developing a Personalized Relapse Prevention Strategy

An individualized relapse prevention plan includes how to avoid triggers and what to do if they are encountered. This strategy should be thorough and include the following elements:

- A list of identified triggers and high-risk situations, along with strategies for avoiding or managing them.

- A schedule for regular participation in supportive activities, such as therapy sessions, support group meetings, or wellness activities like exercise or meditation.

- A list of supportive individuals to contact in times of need, such as friends, family, or sponsors.

- An emergency plan for handling unexpected high-risk situations or intense cravings may include a step-by-step guide on what actions to take to remain sober.

Managing Urges and Cravings

Cravings are a normal component of the healing process and may be controlled with proper coping skills. Some solutions include:

- Distraction: Engaging in activities that occupy the mind and body, like going for a walk, reading a book, or playing a musical instrument might give a momentary respite from cravings.

- Mindfulness: Mindfulness practice can help people recognize cravings without acting on them, realizing that these desires are fleeting and will pass.

- Reframing: By perceiving cravings as a symptom of the healing process, it is possible to minimize their severity.

- Delaying: Delaying the choice to take narcotics might allow the hunger to pass and the reasonable mind to return.

- Self-Care: Making sure that fundamental requirements such as sleep, nourishment, and relaxation are satisfied will help to minimize the frequency and intensity of cravings.

Individuals may equip themselves with the tools and information needed to sustain their recovery path by knowing and preparing for the obstacles of relapse.

CHAPTER NINE

Lifestyle Changes for Sustainable Recovery

Addiction rehabilitation requires adopting a new way of life that supports sobriety and well-being in addition to refraining from drugs. This chapter focuses on the lifestyle modifications required for long-term healing.

Creating a Positive Environment

One of the pillars of successful rehabilitation is a supportive environment. This includes surrounding oneself with individuals who support and nourish one's sobriety, as well as establishing a living environment that encourages serenity and optimism. To create a welcoming environment:

- Develop relationships with friends and family members who support and encourage your rehabilitation.
- Participate in support groups on a regular basis to retain a feeling of community and accountability.
- Make your house free of substances and full of reminders of the blessings of sobriety.
- If your present living situation is not favorable to recovery, consider housing options such as sober living houses.

The Routine and Structure Role

Structure and routine are important in healing because they provide stability and predictability.

A scheduled day can assist with the unpredictability that frequently comes with addiction, lowering stress and the possibility of relapse. To build a routine, do the following:

- Establish regular schedules for getting up, eating meals, working or going to school, exercising, and sleeping.
- Make time for self-care activities like therapy, meditation, and writing.
- Make time to meet with a counselor, mentor, or support group on a regular basis.
- Keep track of obligations with a planner or digital calendar and make changes as required.

Interests and Healthy Activities

It is critical in recovery to rediscover hobbies and healthy joys, since these pursuits may bring joy and fulfillment without the use of narcotics. They can also assist in filling the time wasted previously on substance abuse. Include activities and good pleasures:

- Discover new hobbies or reignite old ones, such as painting, music, athletics, or gardening.
- Exercise on a regular basis to improve your mood and reduce stress.
- Learn how to prepare nutritious and tasty meals that are both soothing and good for one's physical health.
- Volunteer or participate in community service to gain a feeling of purpose and connection to others.

Individuals in recovery may create a life that not only promotes sobriety but also improves general well-being by implementing certain lifestyle modifications.

CHAPTER TEN

Holistic and Alternative Therapies

On the road to addiction recovery, holistic and alternative treatments provide a variety of choices that can augment traditional treatment techniques. This chapter examines how different treatments can help with rehabilitation by supporting the mind, body, and soul.

Investigating Holistic Approaches

Holistic treatments are based on the belief that genuine healing takes place when all components of a person's existence are treated. These methods seek to achieve balance and wellness in the physical, emotional, mental, and spiritual spheres. Among the most important holistic therapies are:

- Acupuncture: Acupuncture is a traditional Chinese medical method that stimulates certain places on the body to facilitate healing and can be especially beneficial in controlling withdrawal symptoms and cravings.
- Chiropractic therapy can ease pain, enhance bodily function, and perhaps minimize the need for pain medication by treating spinal and musculoskeletal alignment.
- Herbal Medicine: The use of natural herbs can aid in detoxification and general well-being, but it is critical to speak with a healthcare expert to avoid drug interactions.
- Biofeedback: This approach teaches people how to control physiological processes like heart rate and muscular tension, which can help with stress management and emotional regulation.

The Function of Yoga and Meditation

Yoga and meditation are techniques that have been proven to have significant mental and physical health benefits, making them especially beneficial in the context of addiction rehabilitation.

- Yoga: Yoga uses a mix of physical postures, regulated breathing, and meditation to strengthen the body, quiet the mind, and improve self-awareness. Regular practice can improve flexibility, reduce stress, and promote inner tranquility.
- Meditation: This technique entails concentrating one's thoughts and being intensely aware of the current moment. Meditation can help people in recovery develop mindfulness, or the capacity to notice thoughts and feelings without judgment—a skill that is especially important for dealing with cravings and emotional triggers.

Spirituality in Recovery: Integrating It

Spirituality can be a powerful component of recovery, providing a sense of meaning and connection that transcends individual struggles, whether through organized religion or personal spiritual practices.

Personal Practices: Engaging in daily personal spiritual practices, such as prayer, meditation, or reading spiritual literature, can provide a foundation of strength and holism.

Community: Being a part of a spiritual community can provide a support network of like-minded people who can help with the rehabilitation process.

Service: Many people believe that acts of service and giving back to others can be a spiritually beneficial practice that deepens their own rehabilitation.

Incorporating holistic and alternative treatments into a rehabilitation plan can open up new channels for healing and growth. As with any therapy method, it's crucial to speak with healthcare specialists to confirm that these practices are suitable and supportive of individual recovery objectives.

CHAPTER ELEVEN

Medication-Assisted Treatment (MAT) and Beyond

Medication-assisted treatment (MAT) has evolved as a critical component of the recovery process for many as the profession of addiction treatment continues to advance. This chapter delves into what MAT is, the current dispute over its usage, and how complementary therapies might improve its efficacy.

Understanding MAT

Medication-assisted treatment (MAT) is the use of FDA-approved pharmaceuticals in conjunction with counseling and behavioral treatments to treat drug use disorders on a "whole-patient" basis. MAT drugs are intended to balance brain chemistry, prevent the euphoric effects of alcohol and opioids, reduce physiological cravings, and maintain bodily functioning while minimizing the negative consequences of the abused substance. MAT has mostly been used to treat opiate use disorder, but it is also used to treat alcohol use disorder and nicotine addiction.

Methadone, buprenorphine, and naltrexone are common opioid addiction medications used in MAT. The principal drugs for alcohol addiction are naltrexone, acamprosate, and disulfiram. These drugs are not intended to be a cure for addiction, but rather to be taken in conjunction with a complete treatment plan that includes psychological and social assistance.

The MAT Controversy

MAT is not without debate, despite its demonstrated usefulness. Some believe that it just replaces one addiction with another, whilst supporters contend that the drugs are tools that when used appropriately, do not produce a new addiction but rather manage the condition of addiction and help patients to reclaim a productive life.

Concerns concerning accessibility have also been raised, since certain places may not have enough clinicians who are skilled and ready to give MAT drugs. There is also debate regarding how long people should be on MAT, with perspectives ranging from the assumption that therapy should be short-term to the belief that certain patients may need to be on MAT perpetually, comparable to the treatment of other chronic diseases.

MAT and Complementary Therapies

MAT is frequently paired with complementary therapies that address other elements of addiction to increase its effectiveness. This comprehensive approach may include:

- CBT (Cognitive-Behavioral Therapy): Assists patients in engaging in the treatment process, altering their attitudes and behaviors around drug use, and building positive life skills.

- Contingency Management: Offers real benefits for being sober, which can help sustain beneficial behavior changes.

- Peer Support Groups: give a group of people who are going through similar things and can give empathy, insight, and accountability.

Mindfulness and stress management techniques, exercise and nutritional assistance, and family therapy, which can help repair and rebuild relationships damaged by addiction, are examples of complementary treatments.

Finally, when combined with thorough treatment and support, Medication-assisted treatment may be a valuable aid in the recovery process.

CHAPTER TWELVE

Long-Term Recovery and Growth

Addiction recovery is a lifetime struggle that goes far beyond the early phases of sobriety. Chapter 12 dives into the notion of success in recovery, the continuous process of post-addiction personal development, and the significance of giving back to others as a component of long-term growth and healing.

Defining Recovery Success

Recovery success is a personal and developing idea. It entails more than just abstaining from substances; it also includes improved quality of life, health, and performance. This chapter addresses how individuals may define their own success by defining and attaining meaningful objectives for themselves. It might include:

- Maintaining physical and mental health - Establishing and fostering good relationships - Achieving job and financial stability

- Increasing self-esteem and personal fulfillment

Success is also assessed by one's capacity to deal with life's obstacles without succumbing to drug abuse, as well as the level of happiness and contentment one feels on a daily basis.

Post-Addiction Personal Development

The rehabilitation path provides a chance for substantial personal improvement. This portion of the chapter looks at how people can continue to grow and change once the initial period of addiction therapy is over. The following are key areas of emphasis:

- Continuing Education: Developing new skills or finishing educational objectives can boost self-esteem and open doors to new possibilities.

- Career Advancement: Recovery can provide you with the steadiness and clarity you need to pursue new career objectives or grow in your existing job.

- Health and Wellness: Maintaining physical health via food, exercise, and medical treatment is essential for long-term healing.

- Emotional Resilience: Long-term sobriety requires the development of coping techniques for stress and emotional problems.

Helping Others and Giving Back

One of the most rewarding elements of long-term recovery might be the ability to help others who are suffering from addiction. This chapter discusses how service to others may help to reaffirm one's own recovery while also offering hope and support to others who are still struggling with addiction.

- Peer Support: Becoming a sponsor or mentor to others in recovery programs may provide vital insight and support.

- Volunteering: Contributing time and resources to rehabilitation clinics, community organizations, or advocacy organizations.

- Telling Your Story: Sharing your story at recovery meetings or public events may both inspire and educate others about the prospects of recovery.

Individuals may establish a satisfying life in recovery distinguished by growth, contribution, and a profound sense of purpose by defining personal success, seeking continual improvement, and giving back to the community.

CONCLUSION

A Vision for the Future

As we near the end of "Mastering Recovery from Addiction: Building Resilience and Understanding the Brain to Overcome Addiction," it is critical to look ahead with optimism and possibilities. As we have seen, the road to recovery is not a straight line, but rather a complex process that unfolds individually for each individual. The future of addiction therapy takes these complications into account, providing tailored and compassionate care that addresses the diverse nature of addiction.

The vision for the future of recovery is based on the concept that addiction is a curable disorder rather than a moral flaw. Addiction stigma must continue to be destroyed so that more individuals feel encouraged to seek help without fear of being judged. As society's view evolves, the aim is that access to effective treatment will increase, and the entire range of recovery alternatives will be available to everyone who requires them, regardless of their circumstances.

As we develop a better knowledge of the brain's role in addiction, advances in neuroscience offer more tailored and effective therapies. This understanding will also serve to improve preventative methods, reducing the burden of drug use problems on future generations.

The combination of holistic methods, which recognizes that effective healing frequently necessitates attention to the body, mind, and spirit also holds promise for the future of rehabilitation. Individuals in recovery might find the particular combination of assistance that works best for them by combining standard treatments with complementary therapies.

Technology plays a supportive role in this goal, with digital tools and resources making rehabilitation more accessible. Technology, from telemedicine services to online support networks, may overcome care gaps and establish relationships that strengthen the recovery path.

Education will remain a cornerstone of the recovery's future. We can build a more educated and compassionate society by educating healthcare practitioners, lawmakers, and the general public about the reality of addiction and recovery. This entails continual research into the most successful treatment techniques as well as disseminating this information to people on the front lines of care.

Above all, the healing future is one of empowerment. It is a future in which people are helped to recover their lives from addiction, build resilience, and discover a sense of purpose and meaning. It is a world in which each rehabilitation milestone is celebrated, acknowledging that each stride forward is an act of courage and fortitude.

We recognize the difficulties that lie ahead, but also the boundless opportunity for transformation and progress as we anticipate the future. The road to recovery is paved with optimism, and it is this hope that will guide people and communities as they strive for a brighter, substance-free future.